Smoothies For Weight loss

Healthy Smoothie 14 Day Plan to

Lose 10kg of Weight, Detoxify, Fight

Disease, and Live Long

Table of Contents

Introduction

Sometimes in life a small change can make a huge difference! Often that small change is the catalyst you need to snowball your way to success. There is no better diet that will give you great results, make you feel good and give you a kick start into a healthier lifestyle than a green smoothie challenge. Green smoothies would possibly be one of the healthiest food combinations, not to mention tastiest! By drinking smoothies you'll find a new you, you never thought you had! It will re-energies you in ways you never imagined! We trust by the time your done with this book will not only be able to make some mean smoothies, you'll also feel and look great in the process! If you simply reading this book for some great and tasty healthy smoothies that great. We have over 50 smoothies recipes ready to go! If you're wanting to start a detox then we can guide you through the stages and if your wanting to lose weight even better this is the perfect book for you!

The most common thing that deters people from finishing a full body detox is the guided knowledge of what to expect and how it all works. And if your reading this book to also lose some weight

I know the pains of trying to lose weight and live a healthy lifestyle. A huge reason people can't maintain a healthy lifestyle is because of a lack of health and nutritional knowledge, a lack of seeing physical results (even after months of trying to eat healthy and sweating it out in the gym) and the worst of all – most people that go on a "diets", starve them self only to buckle to their cravings falling right back into their old habits; even to put more weight back on! Within this book we go through all these points addressing them so you to can live a healthier and energized lifestyle through healthy Green Smoothies!

The first thing we did was put together the perfect 14 day diet to kick start your new healthy eating lifestyle! Then we went on to make sure you understand how to live a healthy lifestyle even after finishing this diet! Before we go any further I want to tell you a little about myself. My name is James Ryan and I remember knowing nothing about smoothies and healthy eating little under a year ago, now I'm an expert! It wasn't always like this though and I certainly didn't become an expert overnight!

It all started when I looked in the mirror and I wasn't happy with what I saw back at me. I also didn't feel good, I never had energy and I never felt good after my meals. I lived a busy lifestyle and didn't have time to even think about a healthy diet let alone try to understand the inns and outs of living a healthy lifestyle. So a friend of mine gave me some advice, he said why don't you just start with one thing "start small" he said. Try and change one thing about your diet and health every week!

So that what's I did and I did it by doing two things! I replaced one meal with a smoothie each day and I only cooked clean low calorie meals! For those of you who don't understand how and why that helped me become a fit and healthier person in the year to come, I will explain..

My friend not only gave me the advice to start small but he also introduced me to the concept of "calorie in calories out"- what's that you ask? Don't worry we will explain that in the next chapter! But for now understand that the easiest way to start a healthy lifestyle and feel better is to just start. So this book will introduce you to some healthy new smoothies as well as give you a 14 day diet plane to not only kick start your new lifestyle but help you lose up to 10kg in weight all through yummy and healthy smoothies! If your not wanting to lose weight bus just want to experiment with some new smoothies that great to we have heaps of smoothies in the following chapters!

Once I personally understood the principle of "calories in calories out" it made my dieting so easy. It also made food fun again and it will do the same for your new challenge. Not only will it make this smoothie challenge a piece of cake it will make the rest of your healthy living habits a synch as well!

As a word of warning it easy to skip the calories in, calories out chapter and go straight to the menu but just in remember this, you'll statistically be more likely to finish something when you understand the reason you're doing it. If you already know about our "calories in, calories out" method; it might actually pay to have another read! You never know, you might learn something new...

Chapter 1: Calories In, Calories Out! (the best way to lose weight)

Calories in, calories out?

What do you mean calories in, calories out?

Imagine your body was a balloon. If you pump more air in, that you let out. What will the balloon do? It will expand, of course. Vice versa, what will happen if you let more air out than you let in? It will contract! Your body is similar but instead of "air" going in and out causing you to expand (put weight on) and then contract (lose weight), its "calories"!

It's the simplest way to lose weight - consuming less calories than your body needs to maintain its original weight.

What exactly are calories...? Every food you consume has calories but some foods have more calories than others! So for example, a of slice cheesecake will have way more calories than apple. But a slice cheesecake will have the same calorie intake as a healthy sub from Subway. One is simply bigger and more filling than the other – the subway of course.

So if that's case why can't I just eat a cheese cake for lunch instead of the Sub? Cheesecakes taste way better right!? Well you can but do you think you'll still be hungry after a cheese cake. The answer to that is yes. So after eating a cheesecake you'll be more than likely to eat more food thus increasing your daily calorie intake. So the trick to dieting and losing weight is consuming food that fill you up and has a low calorie intake.

Before we go on any further, I'll explain what is meant by "maintain original weight". So imagine the balloon again. But when you're putting air in (calories in) there is a whole on the other end slowly letting air out (calories out). So the balloon never goes up or down, it just stays the same size. Now your body, in a usual day with no exercise needs to burn calories (that's the hole on the other end of the balloon) - to make energy for you to go about your day. Much like a car uses fuel to go from A to B. So you're naturally burning calories throughout the day. The bigger you are, the more calories you will need to burn to keep your body moving. Much like a smaller car burns through less fuel than a bigger car.

So you're probably asking, if I burn calories naturally why don't I lose weight naturally? Well it's simple! Most people either overeat, eat food with high calorie intake or both!

So for example if you were a 28 old female and weighed 222 pounds doing no exercise at all, you'd have to eat 2263 calories to maintain your current weight. If you were to however eat under that amount you would evidently lose weight! That's why when you restrict your calorie intake, you lose weight. Simply put, your body starts using the fat stored to make energy and keep your body alive. When you're eating less calories than your body needs to maintain its current weight.

So why is it that people who starve themselves and lose weight then put a whole heap of weight back on once they go off their diet? It's simple! BECAUSE THEY OVEREAT! As well as that, most people haven't kicked their bad habits that they started with (e.g. eating greasy fatty food).

Think about this very carefully! If at 222 pounds of weight you had to eat 2263 calories to maintain your weight and then you went on a binge diet and lost 23 pounds what would happen if you continued to eat that much food again. Think back to the balloon analogy, the more air in (calories consumed) then air out (calories burnt) then the balloon is going to expand. The same thing happens to your body.

Now after learning this, do not go and starve yourself! That's the worse and most dangerous thing you can do! Like we said before most people put it back on. Instead of starving yourself, eat what you enjoy! Just keep an eye on the calories. Our recipes will help you do this! Also remember that weight loss and gaining a healthy lifestyle is a marathon and you learn one thing at a time!

If you do however have a question or a complaint, join our Facebook group "healthyhealthylifestyle" it's a great community. The best thing is that everyone can help you count the calories if you're not sure!

The best thing to remember with weight loss is that it's a marathon, not a sprint race! It's best to lose 1 pound at a time! Plus life is too short to be starving all the time! There are too many yummy foods out there!

So why does a green smoothie diet help me consume less calories

It's Simple! Green smoothies fill you up but at the same time have very low calorie intake!

Learning how to work out your maximum and calorie intake

Now, actually working out your calories that you need to consume is a complex thing and within this book our goal is to not complicate you but give you the simplest tools to get the best most effective results! So towards the end of this chapter, we teach you the most effective and simplest way to track and manage your calorie intake! So sit tight!

What about macros and micros

So if you've read anything about fitness and health we are sure you would have heard these terms before. So they must be important right!? Well, yes they are but because our goal is to keep things simple for you every diet plane we subscribe we have already worked out your macro and micro's. We really don't want to confuse you with any confusing science so trust in us and as you continue down your path with Healthy Healthy Lifestyle getting more serious about your health well slowly but surely educate you on your path of healthy living.

Learning about exercise

Do you need to exercise to lose weight? The short answerer is no. Again if you remember weight loss is dictated by the amount of calories that you consume and the amount you burn. If you burn more than you consume you will lose weight! So why do exercise if you don't need to. Well for starters, when you exercise you feel good, you are healthier, you get rid of bad toxins in your body. There are countless reasons why exercise is needed in life. Also, if you exercise then you have burnt more calories which means either you can lose more weight that day OR you can enjoy cheeky cheesecake with your friend for lunch! Just one slice though!

Basically it works like this, if you do exercise you will have burnt more calories meaning you will lose more weight that day BUT it also means you will be more hungry. So you have two choices, you can enjoy more food because we all know; food is life! Or, you can choose not to eat any more and enjoy the peace of mind that you've burnt more calories that day. Fast tracking your weight loss and increasing your health.

But how do I calculate how many calories I'm supposed to eat? We use the point system! And what's the points system you ask? It works like this. A team of experts are placed in charge by the Chief Scientific Officer to determine how many points members need to consider in relation to his/her weight, height, gender, and age.

The equation is calculated to determine the 'member's' resting metabolic rate or the number of calories your body can burn daily. Once that number is discovered, the team focuses on determining how many calories should be consumed daily to lose one to two pounds each week.

All sounds very confusing doesn't it! Scientists... metabolic heart rate... We told you this stuff was confusing. Probably the reason you may be finding it so hard to lose weight in the past.

Don't stress though we have made it super easy for you! Go to this site http://www.healthyweightforum.org/eng/calculators/ww-points-plus and plug in your current weight and height and age it will tell you exactly how many calories you are allowed to eat in a day.

Once you work out the amount of points you can eat in a day simply apply them to the recipes we supply in Chapter 3.

Having said that we have actually haven't added points to these smoothies. All we have done is made sure each smoothie doesn't have any more than 200 calories meaning you can eat up to four a day. We did this to make it even more simpler for you. So no need to worry about any confusing Maths!

Chapter 2: Green smoothie basics and why they are good for you!

We're bombarded by chemicals and toxins every day! Everything from the processed foods you eat, the air you breath even the beauty products you apply to your body! In the ideal world avoiding coming into contact with all these bad stimulate would be great but let's be honest, that's not realistic at all! So our best bet of reducing the harmful toxins out body is by consuming foods that aid in removing them!

A small note, many people like to go on detox challenges to lose weight. We actually have another book explain the process of how to lose weight via healthy smoothies and all the added benefits of it. For more information, visit our site at Healthy Healthy Lifestyle.

Starting your detox there is some symptoms that some people may go through in some cases. Why do you get side effects? Your bodies liver, kidney and to some extent, your lungs, are working overtime constantly ridding your body of toxic substances. A well as this when you go "cold Turkey" on coffee or you cut out all added sugars, or you suddenly remove stimulants like chocolate from your diet, you will be experiencing withdrawal symptoms. This is because sugar, caffeine and other stimulant substances can be very addictive for your body and it will react when it is no longer given these substances

Most of these detox symptoms are caused when people suddenly switch to a raw and or vegan diet. Common detox symptoms include;

Acute acne : This is because you often start absorbing many extra fats through such fruits like avocado which are full of fats (although good ones)

Gas and bloating: Gas and bloating are common symptoms of suddenly increasing fruit and vegetable intake. It should however subside within a few days as your body adjusts to a healthy increase of fruits and vegetables. If they don't however simply cut back a little bit on your detox and let your body adjust.

Diarrhea : When fruit and vegetable consumption is suddenly increased it's a real shock to the body. But don't stress this temporary, and it has nothing to do with detoxification. Once your body adjusts to the the increase in healthy food and fiber, the symptoms will subside.

Fatigue and low energy : As most smoothies don't have many calories the body tends ot get fatigued as your eating less than 1500 calories per day (on a full smoothie detox) The best way to avoid this is to track your calories and if you're feeling a little down eat a little bit of food.

Extreme cravings : Extreme cravings are a commonly reported detox symptom, but they actually have numerous causes, and may not be directly related to detoxification. Agina your body may be be reacting to the withdrawel of sugar or caffine. Often though it because your getting insufficient calories! So again just eat a little bit of "healthy" (not the chocolate your craving) food and you will be fine!

Okay that covers most of the side effects you may get but don't stress! Were just making you aware of some side effects. Most people who start a detox challenge and are completely fine! Plus the benefits of a drinking detoxing smoothies far out ways the negatives!

Smoothie detoxes especially green smoothie detoxes reduce cholesterol, increase energy levels and can even improve your skin acting as a ant- aging cure!

Before I go on to tell you the multiple health benefits of smothies I want to tell you about some research I uncovered. I found a research peace that compared chimpanzees to humans. Did you know that us humans share an estimated 99.4% of our genes with chimpanzees! Crazy right! But unlike humans chimpanzees have extremely strong natural immunity to AIDS, hepatitis C, cancer and other fatal human illnesses. So why is that? Well the article put it down to their diet. Unlike the average American who eats almost 100% cooked or processed food, chimpanzees eat a 100% raw and whole food diet!

Further study taught me that these greens that chimpanzees eat are the cause to there high immune system! Well if that's not enough to get you starting to eat more raw green foods, I don't know what will!

Now the best way to digest these raw greens, to help your body maximize the there nutrients is in liquid form. This is because greens are high in cellulose which makes them difficult for the digestive system to break down. However, in a perfectly healthy human body and with the absence of natural deficiencies (cause by eating to much process food) green are liquefied in two ways. Firstly, by chewing and secondly by being mixed with stomach acid. Unfortunately, due to 99% of the populations diet the average American lacks the hydrochloric acid levels needed to help break down these greens. On top of this most people are in such a hurry in their day to day life they don't even have the time to chew there food properly!

Now, I then started researching the benefits of the greens. Turns out there is a huge difference in green leaves and green vegetables. The vegetables contain a LOT of starch (sugar) which combined with the starchy fruits may cause bloating. Green leaves however, contain heaps of fiber which also helps slow the absorption of sugar in fruit making for a powerful combination!

So now that you understand why there healthy let me tell you what you can find in the average smoothie making it SO good for the body!

Vitamin A:

Vitamin A is important for your vision, the immune system, and reproduction. Vitamin A also helps the heart, lungs, kidneys, and other organs work properly. It also acts as maintenance of teeth, bones, soft tissue, white blood cells, the immune system and mucus membranes. Vitamin A also a antioxidant fighting cell. What doe sthat mean? Antiioxidant are responsible for inhibiting oxidation of molecules which essentially damages cells.

In short it prohibits things like cancer from accuring! Wow that's a lot for one little vitimane!

B vitamins:

What are V vitamins? Well to start with there are 8 of them! B1, B2, B3, B5, B6, B7, B9, B12 — play an important role in keeping our bodies running like well-oiled machines. These essential nutrients help convert our food into fuel, allowing us to stay energized throughout the day

Vitamin C:

This vitamin is great for fighting the common cold! It helps bost your immune system, as well as preventing heart disease. It even helps wounds heal faster! Lastly, it even helps fend of wrinkles! Making you young again! How great is that?!

Vitamin D:

Vitamin D is seen as a vital part of good health and it's important not just for the health of your bones. Recent research is now showing that vitamin D may be important in preventing and treating a number of serious long term health problems.

Besides being full of healthy and much needed vitamins green smoothies also have many, many benefits. Below we list some of the main benefits of a green smoothie diet!

Easily digestible

Studies have proven that vegetables and fruits that have been blended together are naturally healthier than if those same vegetables and fruits were consumed in their natural state. While this might seem counterintuitive, the blending process breaks down the cell walls present in the cells of all plants, making it easier for your body to extract the required nutrients in the process. In a nutshell, the blending process acts as the initial stages of digestion leaving your body free to expend its energy on absorbing as much nutrition from the things that you put into it as possible. As an added bonus, the fiber found in green smoothies also improves digestion overall by forcing your colon to work overtime.

Brimming with nutrition

With 70 percent of every smoothie being made up of healthy greens, it stands to reason that each smoothie you consume is going to run the gamut when it comes to vitamins and minerals. They are also known to contain a dramatically higher concentration of antioxidants and polyphenols which are extremely important when it comes to fighting off degenerative diseases, including cancer. Pound for pound, when compared to juices made from the same raw materials, smoothies contain nearly five times as much fiber as well.

Great replacement for caffeine

While caffeine is a great way to get an extra burst of energy in a short period of time, it is largely void of any real nutritional value. Compare this with the average green smoothie which is so full of vitamins and nutrients that the energy it provides is enough to give a jolt to the system practically on par with a cup of coffee. This makes green smoothies a great way to start the day or to get you through the midafternoon doldrums in style.

Excellent way to detoxify your system
When it comes to initiating a 30-day, 20-day, 7-day or any tiype of detox, green smoothies are a natural choice for flushing your system of a wide variety of toxins. They are so effective thanks to the high amount of chlorophyll that they contain which naturally encourages the cells in the human body to release toxins that they have been holding onto for years, if not decades. The previously mentioned high amounts of fiber also stimulate the colon to ensure it is active for its part of the detoxification process as well.

What's more, it doesn't take a massive amount of green smoothie consumption to begin seeing these benefits either, nor does it require a radical restructuring of your diet beyond simply making a concentrated effort to eat healthy and avoid foods that are naturally high in toxins. For most people two servings of a green smoothie per day is enough to start seeing real results if they keep it up for just a few weeks.

Easy to make and very portable

One of the biggest reasons that many people find themselves unable to maintain a healthy diet is that it can be difficult to find healthy foods on the go. The green smoothie takes care of these concerns as practically all green smoothies can be ready to go in less than 5 minutes and each preparation can easily make 2 or more servings. As long as there is a cool place for storage, most of the smoothies in the following pages will keep for about 24 hours meaning that 5 minutes in the morning is all you need to set yourself up for success for the entire day.

The following chapters contain 7 days worth of meals, breakfasts, lunches, dinners and desserts, chosen with the aim to help you detox your system as effectively as possible while still letting you enjoy food! Isn't that great! And best of all, it helps you to lose weight along the way.

The purpose of these next 7 days is to introduce new clean and detoxified food into your diet as well as smoothies. Within you have three options. Option A is the most extreme and hardest but most beneficial for weight lose as well as a full body detox.

Option B is slightly easier than option A as it allows you to eat whole foods as well mixing and matching with smoothies. Option C is the easiest as it starts by introducing clean food into your diet then as you continue into the second week you can start introducing smoothies into your diet. We will explain in more detail below.

Option A:

This will have you going straight into a 7 day cleans. For 3 to 4 meals a day will consist of only smoothies. This is the hardest and most mentally grueling of the three options but if you can hack it out then you will reek the rewards! This method is so effective because by reducing your self to only smoothies successfully reduce your calorie intake while feeding your body with nutrient rich food perfect for a detox. Firstly the average smoothie only has 200 to 250 calories in it and as we aleatory know from the " calories in, calories out" chapter that a reduction in calories means we, yep you guessed it, lose weight. The second thing you are doing to your body is feeding it a maximum amount much needed nutrients! This will help your body quickly and effectively flush out all the bad toxins in your body!

After you have finished the 7 days you can then go on and start option b as your ongoing diet or even option c if you're sick of smoothies.

Option B:

This option is a mix of smoothies and our set daily meals. You could potentially make this your ongoing diet if it suits you. Some people struggle with just smoothies and consequently get hungry and start eating bad food again because the cravings get to much. To battle this we suggest that you replace one or two of the meals in each day with a smoothie. At the very minimum one. This will allow your body to adjust to the change in your diet.

Option C:

This option is the easiest of the three and if your new to dieting or you have found in the past that changes in your diet don't last and you very quickly fall back into old habits then we highly suggest starting with option C! This option you simply follow our daily meal plan then when you start the second week depending on how your feeling you can either do option A and replace all the meals with smoothies or do option B and replace just some meals with smoothies (we recommended having a smoothie for lunch).

In addition to following the suggested meal plan you should plan on drinking one or two of the smoothies listed in chapter 11 to kick your 30-day detox into high gear. Depending on the option you pick the first 7 days is about creating habits. After the first 7 days depending on how you're feeling you can either stay with your current option or pick one of the other two options. Mix and match them as your please!

But before you so start we have supplied the shopping list you'll need for the following meals below. For smoothie ingredients go to chapter 11 where we have all our green smoothies!

Vegetables

- Avocado (5)

- Red cabbage (1)

- Chili (1)

- Carrots (15)

- Yellow pepper (1)

- Edamame (1.5 c)

- Spearmint leaves (12)

- Cucumber (1)

- Garlic (16 cloves)

- Broccoli (4 heads)

- Red bell pepper (9)

- Scallions (19)

- Sun dried tomatoes (1 T)

- Spinach (32 oz)

- Kale (1 c)

- Mushrooms (.25 c)

- Basil (1.5 c)

- Pepperoncino peppers (2)

- Tomatoes (5, 2 lb canned)

- Tomato pesto (.25 c)

- Butternut squash (2)

- Celery (3 stalks)

- Yellow Onion (1)

- Vegetable broth (8 c)

- Onion (5)

- Chives (1 bunch)

- Green Beans (1 lb)

- Orange Pepper (1)

- Yellow pepper (1)

- Cauliflower (1 head)

- Corn kernels (3.5 c)

- Cilantro (1 c)

- Cherry Tomatoes (1 c)

- English cucumber (1)

- Green onion (6)

- Baby potatoes (2 lbs)

- Peas (1 cup frozen)

- Black olive tapenade (.75 c)

- Sweet potato (1)

- Sunflower sprouts (1 handful)

Grains

- Quinoa (4.25 c)

- Corn tortilla 6 inch (8)

- Wheat tortilla 7 inch (1)

- Wheat spaghetti (1 lb)

- English muffin (3)

- Whole grain crackers (5)

- Rice noodles (1 lb)

- Steel cut oats (.25 c)

- Rolled oats (1.25 c)

- Rice (1 c)

- Barley (.25 c)

- Farro (.3 c)

Meat

- Chicken breast (2.5 lb)

- Shrimp (1.5 lbs)

- Smoked Salmon (2 oz)

Beans

- White beans (1 can)
- Red lentils (1 can)
- Kidney beans (1 can)
- Black beans (1 can)
- Garbanzo beans (1 can)
- Baked beans (1 can)

Eggs/Dairy

- Egg (24)
- Buttermilk (1 c)
- Plain Greek Yogurt (5 c)
- Sour cream (.25 c)
- Feta Cheese (2 T)
- Vanilla yogurt fat free (24 oz)
- Pecorino Romano cheese (2 T)
- Milk (4 c)
- Paneer (16 oz)
- Soy milk (2.5 c)
- Cheddar cheese (1 oz)

- Mozzarella cheese (16 oz)

- Lemon yogurt (6 oz)

Seasonings/Sweeteners

- Ketchup (2 T)

- Honey (1.25 c)

- Cinnamon (1.75 tsp ground)

- Vanilla extract (2 tsp)

- Ginger (7 inches)

- Rice vinegar (1 c)

- Red pepper flakes (2 T)

- Arrowroot powder (6.5 tsp)

- Soy sauce (1 c)

- Hot sauce (6 oz)

- Salsa (4 T)

- Chicken bone broth (.5 c)

- Cumin (2.5 tsp)

- Vanilla (1 tsp)

- Black pepper (4 T)

- Lime juice (1 T)

- Lemon juice (1 tsp)

- Nutmeg (.75 tsp)

- Peanut butter (.5 c)

- Cardamom (.5 tsp)

- Cloves (3)

- Paprika (3 T)

- Coriander (.5 c)

- Turmeric (1 T)

- Red chili powder (1 tsp)

- Miso (2 T)

- Gingersnap (1)

- Chocolate chips (.25 c)

- Taco seasoning (1 T)

- Maple syrup (3 T)

- Cayenne pepper (2.25 tsp)

- Garam masala (2 tsp)

- Tarragon (.5 tsp)

- Parsley (2 T)

- Mayonnaise (.25 c)

Fruits

- Raspberries (1.5 c)

- Blueberries (2 c)

- Lemon (1)

- Crushed pineapple (1.5 c)

- Cranberries (1 cups)

- Apple Juice (.5 c)

- Goji Berries (.25 c)

Oils/Butter

- Canola oil (3 c)

- Margarine (3 T)

- Sesame Oil (4 T)

- Olive oil (16 T)

- Extra virgin olive oil (4 T)

- Flaxseed oil (4 T)

- Coconut oil (1 T)

Nuts/Seeds

- Walnuts (1 c chopped)

- Sesame seeds (1 T)

- Chia seeds (.5 oz)

- Flax seeds (.5 oz)

- Pomegranate seeds (.5 oz)

- Fenugreek seeds (1 T)

- Almond milk (.3 c)

- Pecans (1.25 c)

- Cashews (.3 c)

- Almonds (2 c)

Baking

- Celtic salt (10 tsp)

- Sea salt (2 tsp)

- Baking soda (2.5 tsp)

- Baking powder (17 T)

- Sugar (2 c)

- Yellow cornmeal (2 c)

- Whole wheat flour (5.25 c)

- All-purpose flour (4.25 c)

- Pancake mix (1.5 c)

- Brown sugar (4 T)

Chapter 3: Day 1

Option A: replace all 4 meals with smoothies

Option B: Replace 1 to 2 meals with smoothies Smoothie

selection for option A or B see chapter 11

Option C: Follow the whole daily meal plan

Breakfast: Fruity, Nutty Pancakes

For this recipe, you will need to set aside 10 minutes for

preparation, 20 minutes of cooking time and the results will

feed 4.

Nutrition Information

255 calories

10 g of protein

387 mg of sodium

5 g of fiber

2 g of fat (saturated)

67 g of carbs

15 g of fat

Ingredients-Pancake Batter

- Whole wheat flour (1.5 c)

- Sugar (6 T)

- Salt (.5 tsp)

- Baking powder (1 T)

- Flour (1.5 c)

- Baking soda (1 tsp)

Ingredients-Pancakes

- Buttermilk (1 c)

- Egg (1)

- Water (.25 c)

- Cinnamon (.25 tsp)

- Banana (1 thinly sliced)

- Canola oil (1 T)

- Pancake mix (1.3 c)

- Raspberries (.5 c)

- Vanilla extract (1 tsp)

- Honey (.3 c)

- Water (1 T)

- Walnuts (.5 c chopped)

Cooking instructions

- Place the cornmeal, both types of flour, baking powder, sugar, baking soda and salt into a mixing bowl and combine thoroughly.
- Take 1.3 c of the results and mix with the cinnamon in a separate bowl.
- In yet another bowl, combine the buttermilk, egg, water, vanilla extract and canola oil and mix thoroughly before adding in the banana slices.
- In a final bowl, combine the walnuts, honey and 1 T water.
- Prepare a skillet before setting it on the stove above a burner set to medium.
- .25 c of batter will make one pancake. Each side of each pancake will need to cook for approximately 2 minutes.
- Top the finished pancakes using the honey mixture and the raspberries.

Lunch: Sesame and Ginger Quinoa Salad

For this recipe, you will need to set aside 10 minutes for preparation, 15 minutes of cooking time and the results will feed 4.

Nutrition Information

363 calories

15 g of protein

197 mg of sodium

8 g of fiber

2 g of fat (saturated)

43 g of carbs

14 g of fat

<u>Ingredients</u>

- Water (2 c)

- Edamame (1.5 c)

- Quinoa (1 c rinsed)

- Salt (.25 tsp)

- Carrots (3 medium diced)

- Chili (.5 diced)

- Yellow pepper (.5 diced)

- Sesame oil (2 T)

- Rice vinegar (2 T)

- Red cabbage (1 c chopped)

- Sesame seeds (1 T)

- Ginger (.4 tsp)

Cooking instructions

- Turn a boiler to a high heat before combining the water, quinoa and salt together in a covered pot and placing the pot on the boiler. After it reaches the boiling point reduce the heat to low and let the quinoa cook 15 minutes or until the water is completely absorbed.

- Combine the peppers, carrots, cabbage, edamame and the quinoa in a bowl and mix well.

- Separately in another bowl, combine the ginger, sesame oil, rice vinegar and sesame seeds together and mix well.

- Combine the two bowls prior to serving.

Dinner: Garlic Chicken with Soy Sauce and Ginger

For this recipe, you will need to set aside 20 minutes for preparation, 12 minutes of cooking time and the results will feed 4.

Nutrition Information

394 calories

51 g of protein

1120 mg of sodium

2.8 g of fiber

1 g of fat (saturated)

25 g of carbs

10.4 g of fat

<u>Ingredients</u>

- Soy sauce (.5 c)

- Arrowroot powder (3.5 tsp)

- Ginger (2 T chopped)

- Water (.5 c)

- Honey (.25 c)

- Broccoli (16 oz)

- Garlic (2 cloves)

- Chicken breast (2 lbs)

- Olive oil (2 T)

- Carrots (4 sliced)

- Red pepper flakes (as needed)

Cooking instructions

- In a small bowl, mixt together the arrowroot powder, water, honey and soy sauce.

- Place the results into a sauce pan before setting the pan above a burner to a medium/low. Allow the sauce 5 minutes to thicken, stir approximately once per minute.

- Set a large skillet above a burner turned to medium/high and coat it with the olive oil. Add in the chicken as well as the carrots stirring regularly and let it cook approximately 7 minutes before adding in the garlic and cooking another minute.

- While waiting for the chicken to cook, microwave the broccoli until it is cooked to your desired level of firmness.

- Once the broccoli has cooked, add the sauce to the skillet and mix well.

- Top with red pepper flakes as desired before serving.

Dessert: Banana Bread with Blueberries

For this recipe, you will need to set aside 10 minutes for preparation, 40 minutes of cooking time and the results will feed 16.

Nutrition Information

197 calories

5 g of protein

134 mg of sodium

2 g of fiber

1 g of fat (saturated)

29 g of carbs

8 g of fat

<u>Ingredients</u>

- Baking soda (.5 tsp)

- Banana (3)

- Avocado (.25 c)

- Sugar (.75 c)

- Baking soda (.5 tsp)

- Salt (1 tsp)

- Whole wheat flour (.5 c)

- Baking powder (1 tsp)

- Whole wheat flour (.5 c)

- Vanilla extract (1 tsp)

- Eggs (3)

- Blueberries (.5 c)

- Water (3 T)

- Margarine (3 T)

Cooking instructions

- Set your oven to 350 degrees F beforehand

- Combine the baking soda and the bananas in a mixing bowl.

- In another bowl, combine the avocado, sugar and margarine before then adding in the eggs one by one.

Next, add in the salt, baking powder, all of the flour and mix enough for the ingredients to begin to combine.

- Combine the two bowls before adding in the water and vanilla, finally fold in the blueberries.
- Add the results to two 8 in loaf pans and let them bake for 40 minutes. The bread is finished when an inserted toothpick comes out clean.
- Cool 5 minutes prior to serving.

Chapter 4: Day 2

Option A: Replace all 4 meals with smoothies

Option B: Replace 1 to 2 meals with smoothies Smoothie

selection for option A or B see chapter 11

Option C: Follow the whole daily meal plan

Breakfast: Huevoes Rancheros with a Spicy Kick

For this recipe, you will need to set aside 10 minutes for

preparation, 16 minutes of cooking time and the results will feed

4.

Nutrition Information

331 calories

16 g of protein

245 mg of sodium

10 g of fiber

3 g of fat (saturated)

42 g of carbs

12 g of fat

Ingredients

- White beans (16 oz)
- Red bell pepper (1 stripped)
- Cumin (1 tsp)
- Scallions (4 sliced)
- Garlic (2 minced cloves)
- Chicken broth (.5 c)
- Plain Greek Yoghurt (4 T)
- Avocado (1 c peeled, sliced)
- Eggs (4)
- Hot sauce (as needed)
- Salsa (4 T)
- Six-inch corn tortillas (8)

Cooking instructions

- Apply cooking spray to your skillet before placing it on the stove above a burner set to a medium/high heat.
- Add the cumin to the skillet and allow it 30 seconds to cook, stirring continuously. Once it becomes fragrant,

mix in the red bell pepper, chicken broth, scallions, garlic and beans.

- Allow the ingredients in the skillet to boil before turning the heat down and letting everything simmer for 8 minutes until the skillet is nearly devoid of broth. Once this occurs mash the beans until the results are lumpy.

- Create 4 separate indentations in the beans before cracking the eggs and adding one to each indentation.

- Place a lid on your skillet and let the eggs cook until they reach the state which you prefer.

- Split the results in the skillet into 4 before topping with the avocado, salsa, yoghurt and hot sauce. Serve with tortillas.

Lunch: Kale and Spinach Feta Wrap

For this recipe, you will need to set aside 10 minutes for preparation, 6 minutes of cooking time and the results will feed 1.

Nutrition Information

252 calories

16.2 g of protein

600 mg of sodium

5 g of fiber

4.5 g of fat (saturated)

23 g of carbs

11 g of fat

Ingredients

- Mushrooms (.25 c sliced)
- Spinach (1 c)
- Feta cheese (2 T)
- Whole wheat tortilla (7 in)
- Black pepper (.25 tsp)
- Kale (1 c)
- Sun dried tomatoes (1 T chopped)
- Egg (1)
- Egg white (1 whisked)

- Warm the tortilla by placing it in the microwave and letting it cook for 1 minute on the standard power setting.

- At the same time, coat a skillet using cooking spray before placing it on the stop above a burner turned to a medium heat. Place the mushrooms into the skillet before seasoning with the pepper and letting them cook for 2 minutes.

- Mix in the spinach and let it cook until it begins to wilt which should take approximately another 2 minutes.

- Mix in the egg and let them cook until they have begun to set which should take approximately 2 more minutes.

- Place the results into the tortilla and top with the feta cheese and chopped sun dried tomato prior to serving.

Dinner: Pasta Topped with Spinach and Homemade Tomato Sauce

For this recipe, you will need to set aside 25 minutes for preparation, 12 minutes of cooking time and the results will feed 4.

Nutrition Information

399 calories

14.5 g of protein

818 mg of sodium

9 g of fiber

4 g of fat (saturated)

41 g of carbs

15.5 g of fat

Ingredients

- Whole wheat spaghetti (1 lb)

- Garlic (4 cloves chopped)

- Fresh spinach (10 oz)

- Pecorino Romano cheese (2 T)

- Tomatoes (4 chopped)

- Dried pepperoncino peppers (2 chopped)

- Sea salt (1 tsp)

- Basil (.5 c chopped)

- Extra virgin olive oil (2.5 T)

Cooking instructions

- Place the pasta into a medium-sized pot and let it cook according to the provided directions

- While the pasta is cooking, place your skillet onto the stove above a burner turned to a medium heat. Coat the skillet using the olive oil before adding in the pepperoncino peppers and letting them cook for 60 seconds before mixing in the garlic and letting the results cook until the garlic begins to smell fragrant but has not yet burned.

- Mix in the tomatoes and let them cook for 10 minutes or until they are fully cooked and a little soft, stir regularly. Top with the cheese and add in the salt before pouring the results into an immersion blender to thoroughly combine the ingredients.

- Add the results back into the skillet and then add in the basil, spinach and pasta.

- Combine well prior to serving.

Dessert: Carrot Cake Muffins

For this recipe, you will need to set aside 10 minutes for preparation, 25 minutes of cooking time and the results will feed 12.

Nutrition Information

209 calories

9 g of protein

226 mg of sodium

1 g of fiber

2 g of fat (saturated)

32 g of carbs

6 g of fat

Ingredients

- Flour (1.25 c)
- Salt (.25 tsp)
- Whole wheat flour (.5 c)
- Cinnamon (1 tsp)
- Baking soda (.25 tsp)
- Baking powder (1 tsp)

- Sour cream (.25 c)

- Cream cheese (.5 c)

- Canola oil (2 T)

- Sugar (2.5 T)

- Vanilla (1 tsp)

- Brown sugar (2.5 T)

- Egg (1)

- Carrots (1 c)

- Pineapple (.5 c crushed)

Cooking instructions

- Set your oven ahead of time to 375 degrees F

- Place muffin cups into a 12-slot muffin tin

- In a small mixing bowl combine the sugar, cream cheese and egg together and mix well before adding in the pineapple as well as the carrots

- In a separate bowl, mix together the sour cream, canola oil, sugar and brown sugar and blend well before mixing in the vanilla.

- Ensure there is space in the dry ingredients for the wet ingredients before coming the two bowls and mixing well. Take care not to overmix.

- Fill the muffin tins with the results, taking care to leave room in each space for the baked muffin to rise.

- Add the tin to the preheated oven and bake for 20 minutes. The muffins will be fully cooked when you can stick a toothpick into the center of the center muffins and it comes out clean.

- Allow the muffins 20 minutes to cool before serving.

Chapter 5: Day 3

Option A: Replace all 4 meals with smoothies

Option B: Replace 1 to 2 meals with smoothies Smoothie

selection for option A or B see chapter 11

Option C: Follow the whole daily meal plan

Breakfast: Tomato Pesto and Eggs Florentine

For this recipe, you will need to set aside 25 minutes for

preparation, 5 minutes of cooking time and the results will feed

4.

Nutrition Information

175 calories

12 g of protein

462 mg of sodium

5 g of fiber

2 g of fat (saturated)

21 g of carbs

6 g of fat

Ingredients

- Spinach (10 oz)

- Plain Greek yoghurt (.5 c)

- Olive oil (1 tsp)

- Vinegar (1 tsp)

- Sun dried tomato pesto (.25 cups)

- Eggs (4 large)

- Black pepper (as needed)

- Salt (1 pinch)

- English muffin (2 toasted)

Cooking instructions

- Use the olive oil to prepare the skillet before adding it to the stove above a burner set to a medium/high heat.

- Add in the spinach and let it cook for approximately 2 minutes until it begins to wilt. Once this happens, add in the tomato pesto along with the Greek yoghurt and mix well. Remove the skillet from the stove.

- Pour 1 in of water into a saucepan before placing the pan on the stove above a burner that is set to a high heat. Let the water boil and then add in the vinegar along with the salt before turning the heat to low.

- Place one of the eggs into a cup and then add it gently to the water, repeating the process with the remaining eggs. Place a lid on the skillet and allow the eggs to simmer for about 5 minutes, shaking the pan once every 1.5 minutes.

- Split the English muffins in two before placing each on a plate before toping it with some of the spinach. Use a slotted spoon to top each muffin with an egg.

- Add what is left into the skillet before combining it with the pesto and yogurt and mix thoroughly prior to topping each muffin with the results.

-

Lunch: Butternut Squash and Lentil Soup

For this recipe, you will need to set aside 5 minutes for preparation, 8 hours of cooking time and the results will feed 8.

Nutrition Information

253 calories

18.3 g of protein

792 mg of sodium

17 g of fiber

0 g of fat (saturated)

41 g of carbs

2 g of fat

Ingredients

- Vegetable broth (8 c)

- Red lentils (2 c)

- Nutmeg (.5 tsp)

- Yellow onion (1 chopped)

- Carrots (3 sliced)

- Butternut squash (3 c diced)

- Garlic (2 cloves minced)

Cooking instructions

- In a slow cooker, add the yellow onion, butternut squash, vegetable broth, red lentils, carrots, garlic and celery.

- Place a lid on the slow cooker before turning it to a low heat and letting it cook for 8 hours. You can also cook the soup for 5 hours if you use a high heat instead.

- The resulting soup can be successfully stored in the refrigerator for approximately 3 days, after that it should be moved to the freezer.

Dinner: Tikka Masala

For this recipe, you will need to set aside 45 minutes for preparation, 20 minutes of cooking time and the results will feed 6.

Nutrition Information

525 calories

19 g of protein

700 mg of sodium

0 g of fiber

1.5 g of fat (saturated)

28 g of carbs

15 g of fat

Ingredients-Gravy

- Sea salt (1 tsp)

- Canned tomatoes (1 lb, chopped)

- Olive oil (3 T)

- Ginger (2 in)

- Water (2 c)

- Carrots (2 chopped)

- Garlic (4 cloves, chopped)

- Red bell pepper (1 chopped)

- Onion (4 chopped)

Ingredients-Masala

- Nutmeg (.25 tsp)

- Paprika (1 T)

- Cardamom (.5 tsp)

- Cloves (3)

- Cinnamon (.5 tsp)

- Cumin (1 T)

- Coriander (1 T)

- Fenugreek seeds (1 T)

- Turmeric (1 T)

Ingredients-Masala

- Red bell peppers (2 chunks)

- Curry gravy (3 c)

- Paneer (16 oz)

- Almond milk (.5 c)

- Red chili powder (1 tsp)

- Plain Greek Yoghurt (.3 c)

- Sea salt (1 tsp)

- Coriander (.3 c chopped)

- Milk (.25 cups)

- Arrowroot powder (.5 tsp)

Cooking instructions

- Add the ingredients for the masala mixture, along with the olive oil to a Dutch oven that is a minimum of 6 quarts and then provide the oven with a medium/low heat.

- Cook the spices for 2 minutes which should be enough for them to start to become fragrant. Add in the garlic along with the ginger and let everything cook for approximately 30 seconds and then add in the onions, red bell pepper and carrots and cook everything for an additional 3 minutes.

- Once all the vegetables have cooked, add in the chopped tomatoes along with the water and let the mixture come to a boil. Once this occurs, turn the heat to low and let it simmer for 30 minutes.

- Add the results to an emersion blender and blend until it takes on the consistency of sauce.

- Separately, combine the red chili powder, sea salt, milk, arrowroot powder and plain Greek yoghurt together in a mixing bowl and, after combining thoroughly, add in 3 cups of curry gravy and mix well.

- Place the results into a pan before adding in the paneer along with the red pepper. All the contents of the pan to boil before turning the heat to medium/low and letting everything cook for 15 minutes.

- Turn off the heat before adding in the coriander prior to serving.

Dessert: Fruit and Seed Medley

For this recipe, you will need to set aside 5 minutes for preparation, 0 minutes of cooking time and the results will feed 1.

Nutrition Information

228 calories

5 g of protein

10 mg of sodium

1 g of fiber

3 g of fat (saturated)

25 g of carbs

13 g of fat

Ingredients

- Pomegranate seeds (.5 oz)

- Flax seeds (.5 oz)

- Dried blueberries (2 T)

- Chia seeds (.5 oz)

Cooking instructions

- Add the chia seeds, dried blueberries, pomegranate seeds and flax seeds together in a small bag and shake well.

- Shake again prior to eating and enjoy.

Chapter 6: Day 4

Option A: Replace all 4 meals with smoothies

Option B: Replace 1 to 2 meals with smoothies Smoothie

selection for option A or B see chapter 11

Option C: Follow the whole daily meal plan

Breakfast: Protein Bomb

For this recipe, you will need to set aside 12 minutes for

preparation, 0 minutes of cooking time and the results will feed

1.

Nutrition Information

206 calories

9 g of protein

237 mg of sodium

1 g of fiber

0 g of fat (saturated)

338 g of carbs

2 g of fat

Ingredients

- Reduced fat cheddar cheese (1 oz)

- Whole grain crackers (5)

- Egg (1)

Cooking instructions

- Place the egg into a small pot before adding in enough cold water to ensure that it is completely submerged in 1 in of cold water.

- Place the pot onto the stove over a burner set to a medium/high heat and allow the water in the pot to come to a boil.

- Once the water has boiled, remove the pot from the stove and allow 10 minutes for it to cool completely before draining the pot.

- Add cold water to a small bowl and dunk the egg in it prior to peeling for an easier time of it.

- Remove the shell from the egg and slice it into 5 bite sized sections. Place each section onto a cracker and top with cheese prior to serving.

Lunch: Stir Fried shrimp

For this recipe, you will need to set aside 30 minutes for preparation, 25 minutes of cooking time and the results will feed 4.

Nutrition Information

292 calories

42.9 g of protein

752 mg of sodium

5 g of fiber

2 g of fat (saturated)

17.5 g of carbs

5.5 g of fat

Ingredients

- Deveined shrimp (1.5 lb peeled)

- Green beans (1 lb)

- Miso (2 T)

- Ginger root (3 in peeled, minced)

- Broccoli (1 head florets)

- Rice wine vinegar (.25 c)

- Chives (1 bunch minced)

- Sesame oil (2 T)

Cooking instructions

- Fill a large pot half full of water and place it on top of the stove over a burner set to a high heat. Allow the water to boil and then add in the green beans along with the broccoli before covering and letting the pot simmer on a low heat for 10 minutes.

- While the pot is simmering, use the sesame oil to coat your skillet and then add in the vinegar, miso, chives and ginger root and placing the skill on top of the stove over a burner set to a medium/low heat.

- Let the ingredients in the skillet cook for 10 minutes prior to adding in the shrimp. Let the shrimp cook for 5 minutes. Once the shrimp begin to curl and turn opaque flip them and cook for another 5 minutes.

- Combine all of the ingredients prior to serving.

Dinner: Cauliflower and Spicy Noodles

For this recipe, you will need to set aside 20 minutes for preparation, 13 minutes of cooking time and the results will feed 4.

Nutrition Information

324 calories

6 g of protein

1037 mg of sodium

4 g of fiber

2 g of fat (saturated)

48 g of carbs

15 g of fat

Ingredients-Sauce

- Rice wine vinegar (2 T)

- Soy sauce (4 T)

- Unrefined sugar (2 T)

- Ketchup (2 T)

- Arrowroot powder (3 tsp)

- Water (.25 cups)

Ingredients-Meal

- Raw cashews (.3 c)

- Garlic (2 cloves minced)

- Yellow pepper (1diced)

- Rice noodles (1 lb)

- Red pepper flakes (1 tsp)

- Olive oil (2 T)

- Orange pepper (1 diced)

- Scallion (5)

- Cauliflower (1 head, florets)

Cooking instructions

- Prepare the noodles as per the instructions on the packaging.

- Using a small bowl, combine the unrefined sugar, .25 cups water, ketchup, arrowroot powder, rice wine vinegar and soy sauce together and mix well.

- Spread the olive oil onto your skillet before place it on the stove on top of a burner set to a medium heat. Add in the cauliflower and let it cook 5 minutes, stirring regularly. Remove the cauliflower from the skillet.

- Place the yellow pepper, red pepper and orange pepper into the skillet and allow them to cook for about 3 minutes before placing the cauliflower back into the skillet and letting everything cook for 5 minutes.

- Add in the ginger, garlic and cashews before letting everything cook for 2 minutes and then adding in the sauce.

- Increase the heat beneath the skillet to high and allow the sauce to thicken for 60 seconds.

- Combine the spring onions with the noodles and top with the sauce prior to serving.

Dessert: Cranberry Scones

For this recipe, you will need to set aside 20 minutes for preparation, 20 minutes of cooking time and the results will feed 8.

Nutrition Information

308 calories

6 g of protein

350 mg of sodium

5 g of fiber

1.5 g of fat (saturated)

38 g of carbs

15 g of fat

Ingredients

- Pecans (1 c chopped)

- Salt (.5 tsp)

- Orange zest (1 tsp grated)

- Canola oil (2 T)

- Unsweetened cranberries (.5 c)

- Baking powder (2 tsp)

- Low fat vanilla yogurt (1.25 cups)

- Baking soda (.5 tsp)

- Whole wheat pastry flour (2 c)

Cooking instructions

- Prepare your oven by heating it to 400 degrees F

- Take a 9 in baking pan and coat it with a cooking spray

- Combine the baking soda, salt, baking powder, whole wheat pastry flour and the pecans in a mixing bowl and mix thoroughly.

- Separately, place the vanilla yogurt, orange zest and oil together and whisk briskly.

- Form a place for the wet ingredients in the bowl of dry ingredients and combine the two bowls before adding in the cranberries and blending just enough for all the ingredients to begin to come together.

- Add the contents of the bowl to the 9 in baking pan and then form 8 triangles from the dough using a sharp knife.

- Place the pan in the oven and let the dough bake for 20 minutes. The scones are ready once you can stick a toothpick through the middle of the middle scone and withdraw it cleanly.

- Allow the scones to cool for 5 minutes before eating.

Chapter 7: Day 5

Option A: Replace all 4 meals with smoothies

Option B: Replace 1 to 2 meals with smoothies Smoothie

selection for option A or B see chapter 11

Option C: Follow the whole daily meal plan

Breakfast: Scallions and Corn Muffins

For this recipe, you will need to set aside 30 minutes for

preparation, 25 minutes of cooking time and the results will feed

4.

Nutrition Information

345 calories

9 g of protein

491 mg of sodium

4 g of fiber

1.5 g of fat (saturated)

47 g of carbs

16 g of fat

Ingredients

- Egg (1)

- Brown sugar (2 tsp)

- Egg whites (2)

- Corn kernels (.75 c)

- Salt (.5 tsp)

- Black pepper (to taste)

- Sea salt (1 pinch)

- Fat free plain Greek Yoghurt (1 c)

- Whole wheat pastry flour (.5 c)

- Red bell pepper (1 chopped)

- Yellow cornmeal (1.5 cups)

- Canola oil (2.5 c +2 T divided)

- Scallions (4 thinly sliced)

Cooking instructions

- Prepare your oven by heating it to 350 degrees F and prepare a muffin tin with muffin cups.

- Add the 2 T of canola oil to a skillet before setting it on top of the stove above a burner set to a medium heat.

- Add the bell pepper to the skillet and allow it to cook for 5 minutes. Add the scallions to the skillet and allow them to cook for 1 minute stirring as needed. Remove the skillet from the stove and allow the contents to cool for 5 minutes.

- While the scallions and bell pepper cook, mix together the flour, baking soda, baking powder, black pepper and cornmeal in a mixing bowl.

- Separately, add the remainder of the canola oil along with the egg, egg whites, yoghurt and sugar to another mixing bowl and whisk well. Add in the corn and the bell pepper before combining the two bowls and folding in the dry ingredients until they begin to get moist.

- Add the resulting concoction to the muffin tin and then place the tin in the oven to allow it to bake for 25 minutes. You will know when the muffins are done when you can stick a toothpick into the middle of the middle muffin and pull it out cleanly.

- Allow the muffins to cool for 5 minutes prior to serving.

Lunch: Kidney Bean Salad with Cucumber, Red Peppers and Corn

For this recipe, you will need to set aside 15 minutes for preparation, 0 minutes of cooking time and the results will feed 4.

Nutrition Information

274 calories

10 g of protein

24 mg of sodium

12 g of fiber

2.3 g of fat (saturated)

38 g of carbs

15 g of fat

Ingredients

- Lime (1)

- Corn (1.25 c)

- Red pepper (1 diced)

- Kidney beans (1 can)

- Salt (as needed)

- Black pepper (as needed)

- English cucumber (1 diced)

- Cilantro (.5 c)

- Avocado (1 peeled, diced)

- Cherry tomatoes (1 c)

Cooking instructions

- Using a salad bowl, combine the kidney beans, cherry tomatoes, cilantro, cucumber, red pepper and corn before adding the lime juice and mixing well.

- Mix in the avocado and season as desired with pepper and salt prior to serving.

Dinner: Spicy Quinoa Casserole

For this recipe, you will need to set aside 20 minutes for preparation, 90 minutes of cooking time and the results will feed 8.

Nutrition Information

601 calories

37.5 g of protein

797 mg of sodium

14 g of fiber

6.5 g of fat (saturated)

82 g of carbs

15 g of fat

Ingredients

- Taco seasoning (1 T)

- Sea salt (1.5 tsp)

- Cilantro (.25 c)

- Mozzarella cheese (16 oz)

- Tomatoes (1 lb chopped)

- Hot water (4 c)

- Green onions (6 chopped)

- Corn kernels (8 oz)

- Black beans (15 oz)

- Quinoa (3 c)

Cooking instructions

- Prepare your oven by heating it to 3350 degrees F.

- Using a 9x13 rectangular baking dish add in the sea sat, cilantro, taco season, tomatoes, green onions, quinoa, hot water, corn kernels and mozzarella cheese.

- Use aluminum foil to cover the dish and place it into the oven to cook for 60 minutes.

- Remove the dish from the oven, uncover it, add the rest of the cheese and place it back in the oven to bake for 30 additional minutes.

- Prepare your broiler and place the pan near it to broil for 2 minutes to allow the top of the casserole to brown.

- Serve hot and enjoy

Dessert: Ginger and Pecan Oatmeal

For this recipe, you will need to set aside 10 minutes for preparation, 5 minutes of cooking time and the results will feed 1.

Nutrition Information

200 calories

6 g of protein

15 mg of sodium

3 g of fiber

2 g of fat (saturated)

30 g of carbs

12 g of fat

Ingredients

- Apple juice (.5 c)
- Steel cut oats (.25 c)
- Grapefruit (.5)
- Pecans (1 T chopped)
- Ginger snap (1 crumbled)

Cooking instructions

- Combine the apple juice along with the water in a small saucepan and set it onto the stove over a burner turned to a high heat and allow it to boil.
- Add the oats to the saucepan before reducing the heat to low and allowing the contents of the pan to simmer for 5 minutes, stirring constantly.
- Allow the oatmeal to sit for 2 minutes prior to topping with the gingersnap and pecans and serving.

Chapter 8: Day 6

Option A: Replace all 4 meals with smoothies

Option B: Replace 1 to 2 meals with smoothies Smoothie

selection for option A or B see chapter 11

Option C: Follow the whole daily meal plan

Breakfast: Oatmeal with Walnuts

For this recipe, you will need to set aside 10 minutes for

preparation, 5 minutes of cooking time and the results will feed

4.

Nutrition Information

353 calories

11 g of protein

70 mg of sodium

6 g of fiber

1.5 g of fat (saturated)

57 g of carbs

12 g of fat

Ingredients

- Rolled oats (1.25 c)

- Walnuts (.5 c chopped)

- Unsweetened dried cranberries (.25 c)

- Milk (2.5 c divided)

- Salt (1 tsp)

- Dried goji berries (.25 c)

- Brown sugar (2 tsp)

- Water (1 c)

- Granny smith apple (1 cored)

- Pear (1 quartered)

Cooking instructions

- Combine 1.5 cups of the milk and the water in a saucepan before adding the saucepan to the stove above a burner that has been turned to a high heat.

- Let the water boil before adding in the oats along with the salt and reducing the heat to medium/low to allow the oats to simmer for 3 minutes. Stir regularly to encourage the oats to soften.

- Add in the pear along with the apple before covering the pan and letting everything simmer for three minutes until the fruit tenderizes. Add in the cranberries along with the goji berries before taking the pan off of the burner and letting it sit, covered, for 60 seconds.

- Split the oatmeal into 4 bowls and cover each with 2 T walnuts, .25 cups milk and .5 tsp sugar.

- Serve hot and enjoy.

Lunch: Avocado and Chicken Salad

For this recipe, you will need to set aside 5 minutes for preparation, 0 minutes of cooking time and the results will feed 1.

Nutrition Information

425 calories

39.6 g of protein

405 mg of sodium

8.5 g of fiber

1 g of fat (saturated)

34 g of carbs

15 g of fat

Ingredients

- Shredded chicken (.75 cups cooked)
- Plain Greek yoghurt (2 T)
- English muffin (1)
- Avocado (.25 peeled, sliced)
- Lemon juice (1 tsp)
- Sunflower sprouts (1 handful)
- Tomato (.25 sliced)

Cooking instructions

- Place the avocado is a small bowl and mash it to form a paste before mixing in the plain Greek yoghurt and the lemon juice.
- Add in the chicken and mix well in order to coat it completely
- Plate the English muffin before topping with the sprouts and the chicken prior to serving.

Dinner: Bean Burger

For this recipe, you will need to set aside 30 minutes for preparation, 30 minutes of cooking time and the results will feed 8.

Nutrition Information

165 calories

4 g of protein

462 mg of sodium

3 g of fiber

1.5 g of fat (saturated)

16.5 g of carbs

10.4 g of fat

Ingredients

- Corn kernels (.5 c)

- Salt (.5 tsp)

- Tomato paste (1 T)

- Paprika (2 tsp)

- Mayonnaise (.25 c)

- Olive oil (4 T)

- Egg (1)

- Basil (1 oz)

- Mayonnaise (.25 c)

- Broth (1 c)

- Baked beans (14 oz)

- Organic farro (.3 c)

Cooking instructions

- Soak the farro overnight to ensure it is easy to cook, drain the water from it prior to cooking.

- Place the broth and the faro into a pot and then place the pot on top of a burner set to a high heat. Once the broth boils, turn the heat to medium/low and let the farro cook for 30 minutes.

- Let the farrow cool before adding all of the ingredients to a mixing bowl and mixing well.

- Form patties from .3 cups of the mixture.

- Add the oil to a skillet before placing the skillet onto a burner turned to a medium heat. Cook the patties for 3 minutes per side.

Dessert: Peanut Butter Bars

For this recipe, you will need to set aside 30 minutes for preparation, 45 seconds of cooking time and the results will feed 6.

Nutrition Information

168 calories

12 g of protein

327 mg of sodium

2 g of fiber

3 g of fat (saturated)

30 g of carbs

16 g of fat

<u>Ingredients</u>

- Cooked rice (1 c)
- Peanut butter (.25 c)
- Maple syrup (2 T)

Cooking instructions

- Add the peanut butter to a bowl that can be microwaved before microwaving it for 45 seconds.

- Combine the maple syrup, rice and peanut butter in a small mixing bowl and mix well.

- Place the peanut butter mixture into an 8x8 glass container and then place the container in the refrigerator to harden for 30 minutes.

- Cut the bars and consume quickly when removed from the refrigerator to prevent the bars from melting.

Chapter 9: Day 7

Option A: Replace all 4 meals with smoothies

Option B: Replace 1 to 2 meals with smoothies

For Smoothie selection for option A or B see chapter 11

Option C: Follow the whole daily meal plan

Breakfast: Smoked Salmon Frittata with Scallions

For this recipe, you will need to set aside 10 minutes for preparation, 15 minutes of cooking time and the results will feed 6.

Nutrition Information

366 calories

10 g of protein

5335 mg of sodium

0 g of fiber

2.5 g of fat (saturated)

1 g of carbs

15 g of fat

Ingredients

- Tarragon (.5 tsp dried)

- Smoked salmon (2 oz)

- Eggs (4)

- Black olive tapenade (.5 c)

- Scallions (6 chopped)

- Water (.25 c)

- Salt (.5 tsp)

- Egg whites (6)

- Extra virgin olive oil (2 tsp)

Cooking instructions

- Prepare your oven by heating it to 350 degrees F.

- Place the olive oil in a skillet and place the skillet on top of a burner turned to a medium heat. Let the oil heat for 25 seconds and then add in the scallions before letting them cook for 2 minutes, stirring regularly.

- In a small bowl, mix together the eggs, egg whites, water, tarragon and salt and whisk well before seasoning with black pepper.

- Add the contents of the bowl to the skillet and then add in the salmon. Cook all of the ingredients for an addition 2 minutes making sure to stir regularly.
- Add the skillet to the oven and bake for 12 minutes
- Place the tapenade on top before serving.

Lunch: Veggie Burger

For this recipe, you will need to set aside 30 minutes for preparation, 15 minutes of cooking time and the results will feed 6.

Nutrition Information

202 calories

7 g of protein

222 mg of sodium

6 g of fiber

1 g of fat (saturated)

30 g of carbs

6 g of fat

Ingredients

- Parsley (2 T)

- Quinoa (.25 c)

- Barley (.25 c)

- Sweet potato (1)

- Cayenne pepper (1 tsp)

- Garbanzo beans (15 oz)

- Black pepper (.5 tsp)

- Cumin (1.5 tsp)

- Salt (.5 tsp)

- Red peppers (1.5)

- Whole wheat flour (2 T)

- Olive oil (2 T)

Cooking instructions

- Prepare your oven by heating it to 400 degrees F

- Place the sweet potato on a baking tray and place the tray in the oven to bake for 45 minutes until it is nice and soft.

- While the sweet potato is baking, place the quinoa and the barely into two different pots filled with boiling water and let both cook for approximately 40 minutes.

- While the potato is roasting, prepare the red peppers and quarter them before placing them in the oven to roast for 15 minutes.

- Remove the sweet potato from the oven and let it cool before adding it, along with the parsley, cayenne pepper, flour, black pepper, cumin, salt and 1 T oil into a food processor and process well.

- Place the results in a mixing bowl before adding in the barley and quinoa after they have cooled.

- Place the remaining oil into a skillet before placing the skillet onto the stove above a burner set to a medium heat.

- Place spoonfuls of the bean mix into the skillet and flatten them into patties. Each side of the patty will require approximately 2 minutes to brown properly.

- Place each patty onto a whole-wheat bun and top with roasted peppers before serving.

Dinner: Samosa Stir Fry

For this recipe, you will need to set aside 10 minutes for preparation, 15 minutes of cooking time and the results will feed 4.

Nutrition Information

308 calories

8.4 g of protein

536 mg of sodium

9 g of fiber

1.1 g of fat (saturated)

39 g of carbs

7.5 g of fat

Ingredients

- Sea salt (1 tsp)

- Onion (1 chopped)

- Ginger (2 T chopped)

- Cilantro (.25 cups chopped)

- Baby potatoes (2 lb)

- Peas (1 cup)

- Coriander (2 tsp)

- Olive oil (2 T)

- Garam masala (2 tsp)

Cooking instructions

- Fill a pot 50 percent of the way full of water before placing it on top of a burner turned to a high heat. After the water boils, add in the potatoes and add extra water if they are not submerged by about an inch of water all the way around. Let them cook on the burner for 10 minutes.

- While the potatoes cook, add the olive oil to a skillet before adding in the ginger along with the onion. After the potatoes finish cooking add them in as well.

- Place the skillet on top of a burner turned to a high/medium heat and all the contents of the skillet to cook for 3 minutes, stirring twice a minute. Mix in the spice, peas and salt before cooking an additional 60 seconds.

- Remove the skillet from the stove, mix in the cilantro and serve.

Dessert: Savory Nut clusters

For this recipe, you will need to set aside 10 minutes for preparation, 10 minutes of cooking time and the results will feed 4.

Nutrition Information

200 calories

6 g of protein

287 mg of sodium

4.5 g of fiber

2 g of fat (saturated)

32 g of carbs

12 g of fat

Ingredients

- Salt (.5 tsp)

- Honey (2.5 T)

- Coconut oil (1 T)

- Raw almonds (2 c)

- Maple syrup (1 T)

- Cayenne pepper (.25 tsp)

- Red pepper flakes (1 tsp)

Cooking instructions

- Prepare your oven by heating it to 350 degrees F
- Using a mixing bowl, combine the honey, maple syrup, almonds, coconut oil, cayenne pepper, salt and red pepper flakes and mix thoroughly to ensure the almonds are well coated.
- Add the almonds to a baking sheet that you have lined with parchment paper before placing the sheet into the oven for 10 minutes. Stir the almonds after 5 minutes to ensure they are well baked.
- Let the almonds cool for 20 minutes to give the glaze time to set prior to serving.

Chapter 10: Green Smoothie Recipes

Ultimate Detox Smoothies

Kombucha and Spinach Smoothie

This recipe can be ready in 5 minutes, makes 1 serving (24 oz.), and will take approximately 45 seconds of blending assuming you are using a blender that is 1000 watts.

Nutrition Information

334 calories

22 g of fat

10 g of fat (saturated)

35 g of carbs

187 mg of sodium

10 g of fiber

18 g of sugar

3 g of protein

Ingredients

- Kale (1 c)

- Coconut oil (.5 T)

- Kombucha (1 c)

- Frozen papaya (.5 c)

- Cinnamon (.5 tsp)

- Spinach (1 c)

- Honey (.5 T)

- Flax seed (1 T)

- Ginger (2 tsp)

Cayenne and Arugula Smoothie

This recipe can be ready in 5 minutes, makes 1 serving (24 oz.), and will take approximately 45 seconds of blending assuming you are using a blender that is 1000 watts.

Nutrition Information

260 calories

2 g of fat

0 g of fat (saturated)

50 g of carbs

50 mg of sodium

13 g of fiber

30 g of sugar

4 g of protein

Ingredients

- Maca (.5 T)

- Flax seed (1 T ground)

- Cayenne pepper (.25 tsp)

- Pear (1 halved)

- Honey (.5 tsp)

- Green apple (1 cored)

- Arugula (.5 c)

- Ginger (.5 tsp)

- Kale (1 c)

- Dandelion greens (1 c)

- Water (1 c)

- Lemon juice (.5 c)

Spicy Hot Smoothie

This recipe can be ready in 5 minutes, makes 1 serving (24 oz.), and will take approximately 45 seconds of blending assuming you are using a blender that is 1000 watts.

Nutrition Information

340 calories

24 g of fat

0 g of fat (saturated)

32 g of carbs

175 mg of sodium

12 g of fiber

15 g of sugar

5 g of protein

<u>Ingredients</u>

- Water (1 c)

- Kale (1 c)

- Frozen blueberries (.5 c)

- Avocado (.5 peeled)

- Coconut oil (.5 T)

- Chia seeds (1 T)

- Honey (.5 T)

- Chili powder (.25 tsp)

- Protein powder (20 g)

- Coconut flakes (1 T)

- Plain Greek yoghurt (.25 c)

- Maca (1 T)

Flax Seed and Kale Smoothie

This recipe can be ready in 5 minutes, makes 1 serving (24 oz.), and will take approximately 45 seconds of blending assuming you are using a blender that is 1000 watts.

Nutrition Information

275 calories

13 g of fat

5 g of fat (saturated)

40 g of carbs

285 mg of sodium

13 g of fiber

17 g of sugar

6 g of protein

Ingredients

- Frozen banana (1 peeled)

- Coconut oil (.5 T)

- Almond milk (1 c)

- Kale (1 c)

- Cinnamon (.25 tsp)

- Coconut flakes (1 T)

- Honey (.5 T)

- Flax seed (1 T)

- Protein powder (20 g)

Cacao and Avocado Smoothie

This recipe can be ready in 5 minutes, makes 1 serving (24 oz.), and will take approximately 45 seconds of blending assuming you are using a blender that is 1000 watts.

Nutrition Information

260 calories

15 g of fat

3 g of fat (saturated)

30 g of carbs

400 mg of sodium

9 g of fiber

17 g of sugar

7 g of protein

Ingredients

- Spirulina powder (1 T)

- Water (1 c)

- Spinach (1 c)

- Avocado (.5 peeled)

- Cinnamon (.25 tsp)

- Cacao powder (.5 T)

- Honey (.5 T)

- Pink Himalayan salt (1 tsp)

- Flax seed (1 T)

- Maca (.5 T)

- Protein powder (20 g)

Watermelon and Turmeric Smoothie

This recipe can be ready in 5 minutes, makes 1 serving (24 oz.), and will take approximately 45 seconds of blending assuming you are using a blender that is 1000 watts.

Nutrition Information

182 calories

1 gram of fat

0 g of fat (saturated)

45 g of carbs

285 mg of sodium

13 g of fiber

25 g of sugar

4 g of protein

Ingredients

- Frozen banana (1 peeled)

- Dandelion greens (1 c chopped)

- Water (.5 c)

- Watermelon (1 cup fresh)

- Cinnamon (.25 tsp)

- Honey (.5 T)

- Line juice (.5 lime)

- Ginger (.5 T)

- Turmeric (.5 tsp)

- Lemon juice (.5 lemons)

Dandelion and Banana Smoothie

This recipe can be ready in 5 minutes, makes 1 serving (24 oz.), and will take approximately 45 seconds of blending assuming you are using a blender that is 1000 watts.

Nutrition Information

230 calories

1 gram of fat

0 g of fat (saturated)

59 g of carbs

55 mg of sodium

10 g of fiber

34 g of sugar

3 g of protein

<u>Ingredients</u>

- Chia seeds (1 T)

- Coconut oil (1 tsp)

- Spinach (.5 c)

- Coconut flakes (1 T)

- Water (1 c)

- Lemon (.5)

- Frozen banana (1 peeled)

- Red apple (1 cored)

- Dandelion greens (.5 c)

Green Tea and Spinach Smoothie

This recipe can be ready in 5 minutes, makes 1 serving (24 oz.), and will take approximately 45 seconds of blending assuming you are using a blender that is 1000 watts.

Nutrition Information

175 calories

5 g of fat

0 g of fat (saturated)

34 g of carbs

76 mg of sodium

4 g of fiber

20 g of sugar

15 g of protein

Ingredients

- Frozen banana (1 peeled)

- Baby spinach (1 c)

- Brewed green tea (1 cup)

- Honey (1 tsp)

- Protein powder (20 g)

- Honey (1 tsp)

Strawberry Arugula Smoothie

This recipe can be ready in 5 minutes, makes 1 serving (24 oz.), and will take approximately 45 seconds of blending assuming you are using a blender that is 1000 watts.

Nutrition Information

174 calories

5 g of fat

0 g of fat (saturated)

33 g of carbs

133 mg of sodium

5 g of fiber

18 g of sugar

2 g of protein

Ingredients

- Frozen banana (1 peeled)

- Arugula (.5 c)

- Frozen strawberries (1 c)

- Water (1 c)

- Spinach (.5 c)

- Sea salt (1 tsp)

- Honey (.5 T)

- Coconut oil (1 tsp)

Kale and Lime Smoothie

This recipe can be ready in 5 minutes, makes 1 serving (24 oz.), and will take approximately 45 seconds of blending assuming you are using a blender that is 1000 watts.

Nutrition Information

191 calories

1 g of fat

0 g of fat (saturated)

50 g of carbs

35 mg of sodium

5 g of fiber

30 g of sugar

3 g of protein

<u>Ingredients</u>

- Lemon (.5 peeled)

- Frozen banana (1 peeled)

- Ginger (.25 inch)

- Water (1 c)

- Pink Himalayan salt (1 tsp)

- Lime (.5 peeled)

- Kale (1 c)

- Honey (1 T)

Mango and Avocado Smoothie

This recipe can be ready in 5 minutes, makes 1 serving (24 oz.), and will take approximately 45 seconds of blending assuming you are using a blender that is 1000 watts.

Nutrition Information

240 calories

15 g of fat

3 g of fat (saturated)

30 g of carbs

285 mg of sodium

10 g of fiber

16 g of sugar

3 g of protein

Ingredients

- Frozen mango (.5 c)
- Spinach (.5 c)
- Honey (.5 T)
- Cinnamon (.5 tsp)
- Flax seed (1 T)

- Avocado (.5 peeled)

- Frozen blueberries (.5 cups)

- Arugula (.5 c)

- Kale (.5 cups)

Dandelion Greens and Mixed Berry Smoothie

This recipe can be ready in 5 minutes, makes 1 serving (24 oz.), and will take approximately 45 seconds of blending assuming you are using a blender that is 1000 watts.

Nutrition Information

270 calories

15 g of fat

9 g of fat (saturated)

36 g of carbs

75 mg of sodium

7 g of fiber

19 g of sugar

18 g of protein

<u>Ingredients</u>

- Honey (.5 T)

- Frozen blackberries (1 c)

- Coconut oil (1 T)

- Flax seed (1 T)

- Frozen banana (1 peeled)

- Cinnamon (.25 tsp)

- Coconut oil (1 T)

- Water (1 c)

- Dandelion greens (1 c)

Baby Spinach and Pear Smoothie

This recipe can be ready in 5 minutes, makes 1 serving (24 oz.), and will take approximately 45 seconds of blending assuming you are using a blender that is 1000 watts.

Nutrition Information

222 calories

8 g of fat

0 g of fat (saturated)

39 g of carbs

24 mg of sodium

8 g of fiber

26 g of sugar

3 g of protein

Ingredients

- Pear (1 peeled)

- Flax seed (1 T)

- Baby spinach (1 c)

- Water (1 c)

- Ginger (.5 tsp)

- Honey (.5 T)

- Water (1 c)

- Flax seed (1 T)

Spicy Spinach Smoothie

This recipe can be ready in 5 minutes, makes 1 serving (24 oz.), and will take approximately 45 seconds of blending assuming you are using a blender that is 1000 watts.

Nutrition Information

170 calories

8 g of fat

1 g of fat (saturated)

28 g of carbs

300 mg of sodium

4 g of fiber

15 g of sugar

2 g of protein

Ingredients

- Frozen banana (1 peeled)
- Coconut oil (.5 T)
- Honey (.5 T)
- Chili powder (.25 tsp)
- Water (1 c)
- Spinach (1 c)
- Cayenne pepper (.25 tsp)
- Flax seed (1 T)

Romaine Lettuce and Ginger Smoothie

This recipe can be ready in 5 minutes, makes 1 serving (32 oz.), and will take approximately 45 seconds of blending assuming you are using a blender that is 1000 watts.

Nutrition Information

135 calories

4 g of fat

0 g of fat (saturated)

60 g of carbs

85 mg of sodium

1 g of fiber

24 g of sugar

9 g of protein

<u>Ingredients</u>

- Romaine lettuce (3 c)

- Ginger (.25 inches)

- Frozen mango (1 pitted)

- Lemons (2 peeled)

- Chia seeds (2 T)

- Spinach (2 c)

- Water (1 c)

Radish and Greens Smoothie

This recipe can be ready in 5 minutes, makes 1 serving (32 oz.), and will take approximately 45 seconds of blending assuming you are using a blender that is 1000 watts.

Nutrition Information

373 calories

2 g of fat

0 g of fat (saturated)

60 g of carbs

35 mg of sodium

15 g of fiber

16 g of sugar

6 g of protein

<u>Ingredients</u>

- Tangerines (2 peeled)

- Radish greens (1.5 c)

- Water (1 c)

- Red apple (1 cored)

- Dandelion greens (1 c)

- Ginger (.5 tsp)

Chard and Banana Smoothie

This recipe can be ready in 5 minutes, makes 1 serving (24 oz.), and will take approximately 45 seconds of blending assuming you are using a blender that is 1000 watts.

Nutrition Information

200 calories

13 g of fat

2 g of fat (saturated)

35 g of carbs

109 mg of sodium

8 g of fiber

22 g of sugar

10 g of protein

<u>Ingredients</u>

- Frozen banana (1 peeled)

- Almond butter (1 T)

- Mixed greens (2 c)

- Almond milk (.5 cups)

Kiwi Celery Smoothie

This recipe can be ready in 5 minutes, makes 1 serving (24 oz.), and will take approximately 45 seconds of blending assuming you are using a blender that is 1000 watts.

Nutrition Information

150 calories

9 g of fat

0 g of fat (saturated)

45 g of carbs

67 mg of sodium

15 g of fiber

22 g of sugar

11 g of protein

<u>Ingredients</u>

- Spinach (2 c)

- Pineapple (.25 cups)

- Kiwi (1 peeled)

- Water (1 c)

- Celery (2 stalks)

- Frozen banana (1)

Spinach and Mixed Berry Smoothie

This recipe can be ready in 5 minutes, makes 1 serving (24 oz.), and will take approximately 45 seconds of blending assuming you are using a blender that is 1000 watts.

Nutrition Information

275 calories

13 g of fat

5 g of fat (saturated)

40 g of carbs

285 mg of sodium

13 g of fiber

17 g of sugar

6 g of protein

Ingredients

- Spinach (2 c)

- Red apple (1 cored)

- Almond milk (1 c)

- Mixed berries (1 c)

Banana, Spinach and Pineapple Smoothie

This recipe can be ready in 5 minutes, makes 1 serving (24 oz.), and will take approximately 45 seconds of blending assuming you are using a blender that is 1000 watts.

Nutrition Information

300 calories

12 g of fat

2 g of fat (saturated)

22 g of carbs

189 mg of sodium

16 g of fiber

28 g of sugar

11 g of protein

Ingredients

- Spinach (2 c)

- Frozen banana (1 peeled)

- Green apple (1 cored)

- Pineapple (1 c)

- Water (1 c)

Chard and Coconut Smoothie

This recipe can be ready in 5 minutes, makes 1 serving (24 oz.), and will take approximately 45 seconds of blending assuming you are using a blender that is 1000 watts.

Nutrition Information

375 calories

12 g of protein

11 g of fat

4 g of fat (saturated)

28 g of carbs

23 g of sugar

9 g of fiber

54 mg of sodium

Ingredients

- Chard (1 c)

- Plain yoghurt (1 c)

- Frozen strawberries (1 c)

- Frozen banana (1 peeled)

Weight loss smoothies

High Protein Pear Smoothie

This recipe can be ready in 5 minutes, makes 1 serving (24 oz.), and will take approximately 45 seconds of blending assuming you are using a blender that is 1000 watts.

Nutrition Information

299 calories

9 g of fiber

27 g of protein

37 g of carbs

595 mg of sodium

6 g of fat

2 g of fat (saturated)

27 g of sugar

Ingredients

- Almond milk (1 c)

- Spinach (1 c)

- Protein powder (20 g)

- Pear (1 cored)

- Matcha tea (.5 tsp)

Orange Smoothie with Spinach

This recipe can be ready in 5 minutes, makes 1 serving (24 oz.), and will take approximately 45 seconds of blending assuming you are using a blender that is 1000 watts.

Nutrition Information

146 calories

36 g of carbs

3 g of fat

25 g of sugar

100 mg of sodium

4 g of protein

6 g of fiber

0 g of fat (saturated)

Ingredients

- Spinach (1 c tightly packed)

- Navel orange (1 peeled)

- Banana (.5 peeled)

- Coconut water (.25 c)

- Ice cubes (6)

- Hemp seed (1 T)

Orange Protein Smoothie with Kale

This recipe can be ready in 5 minutes, makes 1 serving (24 oz.), and will take approximately 45 seconds of blending assuming you are using a blender that is 1000 watts.

Nutrition Information

300 calories

23 g of sugar

7 g of fiber

613 mg of sodium

35 g of carbs

2 g of fat (saturated)

6 g of fat

30 g of protein

Ingredients

- Water (1 c)

- Kale (1 c chopped)

- Protein powder (20 g)

- Spirulina powder (.5 tsp.)

- Navel orange (1 peeled)

- Cinnamon (1 tsp)

- Ginger (1 tsp powdered)

Green Smoothie with Orange and Ginger

This recipe can be ready in 5 minutes, makes 2 servings (48 oz.), and will take approximately 45 seconds of blending assuming you are using a blender that is 1000 watts.

Nutrition Information

300 calories

40 g of carbs

0 g of fat (saturated)

50 mg of sodium

2 g of fat

12 g of fiber

10 g of protein

28 g of sugar

Ingredients

- Spinach (2 c packed tightly)

- Water (1.5 c)

- Romain lettuce (1 c packed tightly)

- Banana (2 peeled)

- Navel orange (2 peeled)

- Cucumber (1 peeled and chopped)

- Ginger (1 inch)

Green Smoothie with Mint and Blueberries

This recipe can be ready in 5 minutes, makes 1 serving (24 oz.), and will take approximately 45 seconds of blending assuming you are using a blender that is 1000 watts.

Nutrition Information

230 calories

50 g of carbs

5 g of protein

11 g of fiber

35 g of sugar

200 mg of sodium

1.5 g of fat

0 g of fat (saturated)

Ingredients

- Blueberries (2 c)

- Spinach (2 c)

- Mint leaves (4 crushed)

- Kiwi (1 peeled)

- Coconut water (1 c)

- Ice (1 c)

Green Smoothie with Kale and Pineapple

This recipe can be ready in 5 minutes, makes 1 serving (24 oz.), and will take approximately 45 seconds of blending assuming you are using a blender that is 1000 watts.

Nutrition Information

350 calories

8 g of fat

19 g of sugar

12 g of fiber

6 g of protein

3 g of fat (saturated)

45 g of carbs

<u>Ingredients</u>

- Kale (1 c)

- Cucumber (1 c)

- Cilantro (1 c)

- Lemon Juice (1 tsp.)

- Avocado (.5 peeled)

Rolled Oats Breakfast Smoothie

This recipe can be ready in 5 minutes, makes 1 serving (24 oz.), and will take approximately 45 seconds of blending assuming you are using a blender that is 1000 watts.

Nutrition Information

260 calories

8 g of fat

16 g of sugar

40 g of carbs

11 g of protein

6 g of fiber

114 mg of sodium

3 g of fat (saturated)

Ingredients

- Milk (.75 c)

- Banana (1)

- Rolled oats (.25 cups uncooked)

- Spinach (2 c tightly packed)

- Flax seed (2 T)

Honeydew Smoothie with Lime

This recipe can be ready in 5 minutes, makes 4 servings (24 oz. each), and will take approximately 45 seconds of blending assuming you are using a blender that is 1000 watts.

Nutrition Information

240 calories

4 g of protein

15 g of carbs

50 mg of sodium

4 g of fat (saturated)

17 g of sugar

4 g of fiber

9 g of fat

Ingredients

- Honeydew (4 c)

- Mint leaves (1 c)

- Coconut milk (.5 c)

- Ice (1 c)

- Lime juice (1 tsp.)

Peaches and Kale Smoothie

This recipe can be ready in 5 minutes, makes 1 serving (24 oz.), and will take approximately 45 seconds of blending assuming you are using a blender that is 1000 watts.

Nutrition Information

400 calories

34 g of sugar

33 g of protein

2 g of fiber

600 mg of sodium

60 g of carbs

2.5 g of fat (saturated)

9 g of fat

Ingredients

- Frozen peaches (1 c)

- Protein powder (20 g)

- Almond milk (1 c)

- Banana (1 peeled)

- Pineapple (1 c frozen)

- Flaxseed (1 T)

- Kale (2 c)

Pineapple Avocado Smoothie

This recipe can be ready in 5 minutes, makes 2 servings (12 oz. each), and will take approximately 45 seconds of blending assuming you are using a blender that is 1000 watts.

Nutrition Information

169 calories

20 g of carbs

6 g of fat

6 g of sugar

18 g of protein

4 g of fiber

0 g of fat (saturated)

345 mg of sodium

Ingredients

- Kale (2 c packed tightly)
- Almond milk (.5 c)
- Pineapple (.5 c chunked)
- Protein powder (20 g)
- Avocado (.5 peeled)
- Ice cubes (1 c)

Agave, Spinach and Kale Smoothie

This recipe can be ready in 5 minutes, makes 2 servings (24 oz. each), and will take approximately 45 seconds of blending assuming you are using a blender that is 1000 watts.

Nutrition Information

300 calories

80 mg of sodium

5 g of protein

40 g of carbs

8 g of fat (saturated)

9 g of fiber

16 g of sugar

15 g of fat

<u>Ingredients</u>

- Coconut milk (.5 c)

- Coconut water (1 c)

- Agave syrup (1 T)

- Pear (1 peeled, cored)

- Lime juice (1 lime)

- Spinach (2 c)

- Kale (2 c)

Spicy Green Smoothie

This recipe can be ready in 5 minutes, makes 1 serving (24 oz.), and will take approximately 45 seconds of blending assuming you are using a blender that is 1000 watts.

Nutrition Information

260 calories

32 g of carbs

14 g of sugar

4 g of fat (saturated)

12 g of fat

125 mg of sodium

8 g of protein

6 g of fiber

Ingredients

- Cayenne pepper (1 tsp)
- Avocado (.5 peeled)
- Coconut water (1 c)
- Kale (1 c)
- Frozen pineapple (.5 c)
- Spinach (1 c)

Honey and Spinach Smoothie

This recipe can be ready in 5 minutes, makes 1 serving (24 oz.), and will take approximately 45 seconds of blending assuming you are using a blender that is 1000 watts.

Nutrition Information

300 calories

4 g of fat

1 g of fiber

45 g of protein

25 g of carbs

19 g of sugar

2 g of fat (saturated)

140 mg of sodium

Ingredients

- Honey (1 T)

- Spinach (1 c)

- Protein powder (20 grams)

- Ice (1 c)

- Ice water (5 oz)

Apple and Greens Smoothie

This recipe can be ready in 5 minutes, makes 1 serving (24 oz.), and will take approximately 45 seconds of blending assuming you are using a blender that is 1000 watts.

Nutrition Information

290 calories

600 mg of sodium

2 g of fat (saturated)

28 g of protein

34 g of carbs

23 g of sugar

7 g of fiber

6 g of fat

Ingredients

- Kale (1 c)
- Spinach (1 c)
- Almond milk (1 c)
- Cucumber (1 chopped)
- Protein powder (20 g)

- Green apple (1 cored)

- Lemon juice (1 tsp)

Avocado and Lime Smoothie

This recipe can be ready in 5 minutes, makes 1 serving (24 oz.), and will take approximately 45 seconds of blending assuming you are using a blender that is 1000 watts.

Nutrition Information

340 calories

10 g of protein

34 g of carbs

19 g of sugar

9 g of fiber

8 g of fat (saturated)

50 mg of sodium

22 g of fat

Ingredients

- Baby spinach (.5 c)

- Lime (1 peeled)

- Lime zest (1 lime)

- Almond milk (1 c)

- Avocado (.5 peeled)

- Vanilla extract (.5 tsp)

- Honey (.5 T)

- Vanilla extract (.5 tsp)

- Sea salt (1 tsp)

Basil and Chlorella Smoothie

This recipe can be ready in 5 minutes, makes 1 serving (24 oz.), and will take approximately 45 seconds of blending assuming you are using a blender that is 1000 watts.

Nutrition Information

320 calories

240 mg of sodium

15 g of fat

10 g of fiber

4 g of fat (saturated

13 g of protein

35 g of carbs

Ingredients

- Frozen pineapple (.5 c chunks)

- Coconut water (1 c)

- Avocado (.5 peeled)

- Basil (6 leaves)

- Plain yoghurt (.25 c)

- Chia seeds (1 tsp)

- Maca (1 tsp)

- Chlorella (1 tsp)

- Lemon juice (1 tsp)

- Bee pollen (1 tsp)

- Sea salt (1 tsp)

- Honey (.5 T)

Berries and Beets Smoothie

This recipe can be ready in 5 minutes, makes 1 serving (24 oz.), and will take approximately 45 seconds of blending assuming you are using a blender that is 1000 watts.

Nutrition Information

280 calories

30 mg of sodium

7 g of fat (saturated)

21 g of sugar

4 g of protein

38 g of carbs

15 g of fiber

15 g of fat

Ingredients

- Coconut oil (1 T)

- Ginger (2 tsp)

- Beet greens (.5 c)

- Beets (.5 c cooked)

- Water (1 c)

- Frozen raspberries (.5 c)

- Lemon (1 peeled)

- Frozen blackberries (.5 c)

Dandelion Smoothie with Lime

This recipe can be ready in 5 minutes, makes 1 serving (24 oz.), and will take approximately 45 seconds of blending assuming you are using a blender that is 1000 watts.

Nutrition Information

190 calories

1 g of fat

43 g of carbs

80 mg of sodium

6 g of fiber

7 g of protein

0 g of fat (saturated)

25 g of sugar

Ingredients

- Lemon juice (1 peeled)

- Frozen banana (1 peeled)

- Water (1 c)

- Spirulina (.5 tsp)

- Dandelion greens (1.5 cups destemmed)

- Chlorella (1 tsp)

- Honey (.5 T)

- Ice cubes (7)

- Pink Himalayan salt (1 tsp)

Avocado and Mango Smoothie

This recipe can be ready in 5 minutes, makes 1 serving (24 oz.), and will take approximately 45 seconds of blending assuming you are using a blender that is 1000 watts.

Nutrition Information

314 calories

16 g of fat

5 g of protein

100 mg of sodium

48 g of carbs

30 g of sugar

3 g of fat (saturated)

11 g of fiber

<u>Ingredients</u>

- Avocado (1 peeled)

- Cilantro (.5 c)

- Water (1 c)

- Frozen mango (1 c)

- Line juice (1 lime)

- Spinach (1 c)

- Ginger (.25 inch)

- Raw honey (.5 T)

Guacamole Smoothie

This recipe can be ready in 5 minutes, makes 1 serving (24 oz.), and will take approximately 45 seconds of blending assuming you are using a blender that is 1000 watts.

Nutrition Information

350 calories

7 g of fat (saturated)

30 g of fat

250 mg of sodium

24 g of carbs

4 g of sugar

15 g of fiber

5 g of protein

Ingredients

- Avocado (1 peeled)

- Tomato (1 c)

- Water (1 c)

- Line juice (.25 c)

- Sea salt (1 tsp)

- Cilantro (.5 c)

Spinach and Strawberry Smoothie

This recipe can be ready in 5 minutes, makes 1 serving (24 oz.), and will take approximately 45 seconds of blending assuming you are using a blender that is 1000 watts.

Nutrition Information

500 calories

200 mg of sodium

8 g of fat (saturated)

15 g of fat

32 g of sugar

45 g of carbs

12 g of protein

13 g of fiber

Ingredients

- Banana (1 peeled)
- Spinach (1 c)
- Almond milk (1.5 c)
- Frozen strawberries (.5 c)
- Plain Greek yogurt (2)
- Frozen mango (.5 c)
- Chia seeds (1 T)
- Bee pollen (1 tsp)
- Coconut oil (1 T)

Cinnamon and Spinach Smoothie

This recipe can be ready in 5 minutes, makes 1 serving (24 oz.), and will take approximately 45 seconds of blending assuming you are using a blender that is 1000 watts.

Nutrition Information

304 calories

105 mg of sodium

15 g of fat

3 g of protein

46 g of carbs

7 g of fiber

20 g of sugar

3 g of fat (saturated)

Ingredients

- Frozen banana (1 peeled)

- Spinach (1 c)

- Water (1 c)

- Frozen blackberries (1 c)

- Basil (5 leaves)

- Cinnamon (.25 tsp)

- Coconut oil (1 T)

- Stevia (1 tsp)

Wheatgrass and Goji Berry Smoothie

This recipe can be ready in 5 minutes, makes 1 serving (24 oz.), and will take approximately 45 seconds of blending assuming you are using a blender that is 1000 watts.

Nutrition Information

500 calories

22 g of fat

15 g of protein

200 mg of sodium

50 g of carbs

29 g of sugar

20 g of fiber

1 gram of fat (saturated)

Ingredients

- Wheatgrass (1 tsp powdered)

- Stevia (1 tsp)

- Coconut oil (1 T)

- Coconut flakes (1 T)

- Maca (1 tsp)

- Dried cranberries (2 T)

- Greek yoghurt (.5 c)

- Goji berries (2 T)

- Kale (.5 c)

- Frozen mango (.5 c)

- Spinach (.5 c)

- Coconut water (1 c)

- Avocado (.5 peeled)

Aloe Vera and Blueberry Smoothie

This recipe can be ready in 5 minutes, makes 1 serving (24 oz.), and will take approximately 45 seconds of blending assuming you are using a blender that is 1000 watts.

Nutrition Information

275 calories

3 g of fat (saturated)

30 g of carbs

7 g of fiber

45 mg of sodium

17 g of fat

3 g of protein

24 g of sugar

Ingredients

- Aloe vera (.5 cups)

- Avocado (.5 peeled)

- Water (1 c)

- Frozen blueberries (.5 c)

- Coconut oil (.5 T)

- Spinach (1 c)

- Pink Himalayan salt (1 T)

- Stevia (.5 tsp)

- Coconut oil (.5 T)

Strawberry Smoothie with Mint

This recipe can be ready in 5 minutes, makes 1 serving (24 oz.), and will take approximately 45 seconds of blending assuming you are using a blender that is 1000 watts.

Nutrition Information

160 calories

20 g of sugar

40 g of carbs

0 g of fat (saturated)

12 g of fiber

3 g of protein

300 mg of sodium

1 g of fat

Ingredients

- Frozen banana (1 peeled)

- Frozen strawberries (1 c)

- Water (1 c)

- Mint leaves (2 c)

- Spinach (1 c)

- Stevia (1 tsp)

Banana and Rosemary Smoothie

This recipe can be ready in 5 minutes, makes 1 serving (24 oz.), and will take approximately 45 seconds of blending assuming you are using a blender that is 1000 watts.

Nutrition Information

200 calories

50 g of carbs

232 mg of sodium

1 gram of fat

29 g of sugar

9 g of fiber

3 g of protein

0 g of fat (saturated)

Ingredients

- Frozen banana (1 peeled)

- Blueberries (1 c)

- Water (1 c)

- Rosemary (2 sprigs)

- Sea salt (1 tsp)

- Stevia (1 tsp)

Beet Greens and Cinnamon Smoothie

This recipe can be ready in 5 minutes, makes 1 serving (24 oz.), and will take approximately 45 seconds of blending assuming you are using a blender that is 1000 watts.

Nutrition Information

200 calories

1 gram of fat

10 g of fiber

75 mg of sodium

25 g of sugar

0 g of fat (saturated)

50 g of carbs

3 g of protein

Ingredients

- Green apple (1 cored)

- Frozen blueberries (.5 c)

- Water (1 c)

- Frozen banana (1 peeled)

- Cinnamon (1 tsp)

- Beet greens (1.5 c)

- Stevia (1 tsp)

Spinach and Mint Smoothie

This recipe can be ready in 5 minutes, makes 1 serving (24 oz.), and will take approximately 45 seconds of blending assuming you are using a blender that is 1000 watts.

Nutrition Information

230 calories

3 g of fat (saturated)

7 g of fiber

75 mg of sodium

23 g of sugar

40 g of carbs

4 g of protein

8 g of fat

Ingredients

- Frozen banana (1 peeled)

- Spinach (1 c)

- Almond milk (1 c)

- Frozen blueberries (1 c)

- Coconut oil (1 T)

- Mint leaves (1 cup)

- Stevia (1 tsp)

Kale Smoothie with Blueberries

This recipe can be ready in 5 minutes, makes 1 serving (24 oz.), and will take approximately 45 seconds of blending assuming you are using a blender that is 1000 watts.

Nutrition Information

367 calories

13 g of fat

75 mg of sodium

25 g of sugar

50 g of carbs

10 g of fiber

20 g of protein

6 g of fat (saturated)

Ingredients

- Frozen blueberries (.5 c)

- Almond milk (1 c)

- Frozen banana (1 peeled)

- Cinnamon (.5 tsp)

- Kale (1 c)

- Stevia (1 tsp)

- Coconut oil (1 T)

Banana and Beets Smoothie

This recipe can be ready in 5 minutes, makes 1 serving (24 oz.), and will take approximately 45 seconds of blending assuming you are using a blender that is 1000 watts.

Nutrition Information

150 calories

3 g of fat

10 g of fiber

25 g of sugar

75 mg of sodium

0 g of fat (saturated)

50 g of carbs

3 g of protein

Ingredients

- Beet greens (1 c chopped)

- Frozen banana (1 peeled)

- Chia seeds (1 T)

- Water (1 c)

- Coconut oil (1 T)

- Stevia (1 tsp)

Mixed Berry and Lettuce Smoothie

This recipe can be ready in 5 minutes, makes 1 serving (24 oz.), and will take approximately 45 seconds of blending assuming you are using a blender that is 1000 watts.

Nutrition Information

190 calories

0 g of fat (saturated)

45 g of carbs

8 g of fiber

25 g of sugar

210 mg of sodium

4 g of protein

1 gram of fat

Ingredients

- Red apple (1 cored)
- Cinnamon (.25 tsp)
- Kale (1 cup)
- Water (1 cup)
- Pink Himalayan salt (1 tsp)

- Frozen banana (1 peeled)

- Stevia (1 tsp)

Greens on Greens Smoothie

This recipe can be ready in 5 minutes, makes 1 serving (24 oz.), and will take approximately 45 seconds of blending assuming you are using a blender that is 1000 watts.

Nutrition Information

140 calories

15 g of sugar

2 g of fat

4 g of protein

35 g of carbs

150 mg of sodium

4 g of fiber

0 g of fat (saturated)

<u>Ingredients</u>

- Kale (1 c)

- Baby spinach (1 c)

- Coconut flakes (.25 cups)

- Frozen banana (1 peeled)

- Water (1 c)

- Coconut oil (1 T)

Apples, Apples, Apples Green Smoothie

This recipe can be ready in 5 minutes, makes 1 serving (24 oz.), and will take approximately 45 seconds of blending assuming you are using a blender that is 1000 watts.

Nutrition Information

300 calories

32 g of sugar

9 g of fiber

1 gram of fat (saturated)

300 mg of sodium

60 g of carbs

3 g of protein

5 g of fat

<u>Ingredients</u>

- Red apple (1 cored)

- Green apple (1 cored)

- Yellow apple (1 cored)

- Coconut oil (1 T)

- Baby spinach (1 c)

- Cinnamon (.5 tsp)

- Water (1 c)

- Maca (.5 T)

Banana and Mint Smoothie

This recipe can be ready in 5 minutes, makes 1 serving (24 oz.), and will take approximately 45 seconds of blending assuming you are using a blender that is 1000 watts.

Nutrition Information

280 calories

25 g of sugar

6 g of fiber

0 g of fat (saturated)

75 mg of sodium

35 g of carbs

10 g of protein

12 g of fat

Ingredients

- Frozen blueberries (1 c)

- Chia seeds (1 T)

- Almond milk (1 c)

- Mint leaves (10)

- Frozen banana (1 peeled)

- Water (1 c)

- Stevia (1 tsp)

- Coconut oil (1 T)

Strawberry and Salad Smoothie

This recipe can be ready in 5 minutes, makes 1 serving (24 oz.), and will take approximately 45 seconds of blending assuming you are using a blender that is 1000 watts.

Nutrition Information

200 calories

125 mg of sodium

6 g of fat

7 g of fiber

20 g of sugar

40 g of carbs

0 g of fat (saturated)

3 g of protein

Ingredients

- Frozen strawberries (1 c)

- Sea salt (1 tsp)

- Flax seed (1 T)

- Salad greens (1 c)

- Water (1 c)

- Kale (.5 c)

- Cinnamon (1 tsp)

- Frozen banana (1 peeled)

- Stevia (1 tsp)

- Coconut oil (1 T)

Banana and Romaine Lettuce Smoothie

This recipe can be ready in 5 minutes, makes 1 serving (24 oz.), and will take approximately 45 seconds of blending assuming you are using a blender that is 1000 watts.

Nutrition Information

160 calories

0 g of fat (saturated)

6 g of fiber

3 g of protein

40 g of carbs

1 g of fat

20 g of sugar

289 mg of sodium

Ingredients

- Frozen pineapple (.5 c)

- Frozen mango (.5 c)

- Romaine lettuce (2 c chopped)

- Chia seeds (1 T)

- Water (1 c)

- Coconut flakes (1 T)

- Coconut oil (1 T)

- Stevia (1 tsp)

- Frozen banana (1 peeled)

Kiwi and Spinach Smoothie

This recipe can be ready in 5 minutes, makes 1 serving (24 oz.), and will take approximately 45 seconds of blending assuming you are using a blender that is 1000 watts.

Nutrition Information

150 calories

25 g of sugar

0 g of fat (saturated)

3 g of protein

50 g of carbs

75 mg of sodium

3 g of fat

10 g of fiber

<u>Ingredients</u>

- Frozen banana (1 peeled)

- Spinach (1 c)

- Pink Himalayan salt (1 tsp)

- Kiwi (2 peeled)

- Chia seeds (1 T)

- Water (1 c)

- Coconut flakes (1 T)

- Coconut oil (1 T)

- Stevia (1 tsp)

Kale and Green Apple Smoothie

This recipe can be ready in 5 minutes, makes 1 serving (24 oz.), and will take approximately 45 seconds of blending assuming you are using a blender that is 1000 watts.

Nutrition Information

250 calories

6 g of fat

10 g of fiber

55 g of carbs

324 mg of sodium

9 g of protein

0 g of fat (saturated)

29 g of sugar

Ingredients

- Dandelion greens (1 c)

- Water (1 c)

- Spinach (1 c)

- Beet greens (1 c)

- Kale (1 c)

- Coconut oil (1 T)

- Green apple (1 cored)

- Stevia (1 tsp)

Kombucha, Cinnamon and Kale Smoothie

This recipe can be ready in 5 minutes, makes 1 serving (24 oz.), and will take approximately 45 seconds of blending assuming you are using a blender that is 1000 watts.

Nutrition Information

334 calories

10 g of fat (saturated)

35 g of carbs

18 g of sugar

22 g of fat

10 g of fiber

3 g of protein

187 mg of sodium

Ingredients

- Kale (1 c)

- Coconut oil (.5 T)

- Kombucha (1 c)

- Frozen papaya (.5 c)

- Cinnamon (.5 tsp)

- Spinach (1 c)

- Honey (.5 T)

- Flax seed (1 T)

- Ginger (2 tsp)

Conclusion

Thanks for reading our book *Healthy Smoothies: Healthy Green Smoothie 14 Day Plan to Lose Weight, Detoxify, Fight Disease, and Live Long*. And Remember that starting your healthy lifestyle doesn't have to be hard. You now have some powerful knowledge so don't waste it!

The beauty of this challenge is you have now learnt two skills that will help you along becoming a healthier person. The first, making healthy and tasty smoothies and the second, making appetizing and healthy breakfast, lunch, dinners and deserts!

I really hoped you enjoyed my books and if you did please have a look at our other challengers! There great to do every 30 days which means you get to stay healthy and not even have to think about it!

Again thank you for reading and if this book helped you any way at all please feel welcome to leave us a good review!

Description:

If you have been trying to lose weight with no to little success. If you think that it's just to hard or "it's just never going to work for you". Then you are in the right place!

Our scientifically proven smoothie based diet is a proven and tested diet plan that works for everybody and anybody! For most people they struggle to lose weight because they don't plan! The other main reason is that they don't have a understanding of how to actually lose weight.

This book not only has the a menu plan that will help you lose weight it also outlines and explains the process. It statiscaly prove that your more likely to successfully complete a diet plan when you understand it. If your worried about trying to understand fitness jargon, don't stress we have made it so simple to understand that anyone can follow it!

Following this receipe book you can be sure to lose weight, improve your metabolism, gain energy and increase your overall health!

Rest assure if you follow this simple and easy smoothie diet plan you can lose up to 10kg in a little over 2 weeks!

Here Is A Preview Of What You'll Learn...

- Proven and affordable smoothie recipes
- How to get the most out of your diet
- Foods to avoid when trying to lose weight
- 30 different smoothie recipes for weight loss
- Smoothie recipes for more energy
- Easy and simple explanations, explaining how to increase your overall health
- Much, much more!

Download your copy today!
Take action today and download this book for a limited time discount of only $2.99! Its time for you to finally shed that weight while enjoying delicious, and healthy smoothies.